Malek Zribi
Jaweher Kammoun
Samir Maatoug

Forensic evaluation of medical death certificates

Malek Zribi
Jaweher Kammoun
Samir Maatoug

Forensic evaluation of medical death certificates

ScienciaScripts

Cover image: www.ingimage.com

This book is a translation from the original published under ISBN 978-613-8-43142-8.

Publisher:
Sciencia Scripts
is a trademark of
Dodo Books Indian Ocean Ltd., member of the OmniScriptum S.R.L Publishing group
str. A.Russo 15, of. 61, Chisinau-2068, Republic of Moldova Europe
Printed at: see last page
ISBN: 978-620-4-07015-5

INTRODUCTION

The medical death certificate (MDC) is an official document certifying the death of a person. This certificate has its origins in antiquity. Indeed, since this period of history we find traces of attempts to count deaths: in Egypt and Mesopotamia from the 3rd millennium BC, in China and among the Hebrews at the end of the 1st millennium and in Rome in the 6th century BC [1]. In modern times in Europe, the counting of deaths began in England in 1540 for plague epidemics, and was later extended to other causes of death in 1590 [1]. It was not until 1802, in France, that a form was introduced for the certification of causes of death: the ancestor of the medical certificate of causes of death, and the obligation at that time for practitioners to use this form for the declaration of deaths [1]. In 1945, when WHO was created, it was entrusted with the evolution and updating of the classification of causes of death (ICD). This model was adopted in Tunisia by decree n°99-1043 of 17 May 1999 [2]. The CMD, established by a physician, is indispensable for the declaration of death to the civil status services. Indeed, the responsibility of establishing the death falls clinically on the doctor, and legally on the civil registrar. The drafting of the CMD is an indispensable act before any funeral operations. Depending on the circumstances of the death, it can be the starting point for a judicial inquiry. The CMD is not a simple medical formality, it is essential and represents at the same time a civil status act, a social act, a medico-legal act and a source of epidemiological data. The drafting of a CMD requires a precise methodology in terms of its form and content. Legal consequences may or may not follow from this drafting. Despite the teaching of CMD writing rules during medical studies and the presence of writing guides developed by international and national organizations, the various studies show that the frequency of writing errors is still high and is estimated at between 16 and 78% of CMDs [3-8]. The reasons given by the authors are different and multiple and sometimes remain obscure [3-9]. For this reason, it seemed necessary to us to carry out this work aimed at analysing the CMDs. We carried out a study on the CMDs received by the Legal Medicine Department of Sfax with the following objectives

- Review the content of CMDs and assess the quality of the writing;
- Analyze writing errors and classify them as minor or major errors.
- To propose practical recommendations for the establishment of CMDs in order to improve the training of certifying physicians.

MATERIALS AND METHODS

1. TYPE OF STUDY

We conducted a prospective and descriptive study, extended over a period of one year from January [1], 2020 to December 31, 2020, including medical death certificates received at the Forensic Medicine Department of Habib Bourguiba Hospital in Sfax. All cases of sudden death, violent death and suspicious death must undergo a forensic autopsy in order to determine the cause and circumstances of death.

2. DATA COLLECTION

The data were collected using a data sheet (canvas) designed for this study (Appendix 1).

It has two components:

A component to collect :

There are nine types of information about the deceased:

1. Full name ;
2. National identity card (NIC) number ;
3. Address;
4. Age;
5. Gender;
6. Profession;
7. Marital status ;
8. Nationality;
9. Place of death.

Concerning the doctor, there are seven of them:

1. Name;
2. Specialty;
3. Grade;
4. Registration number with the National Medical Council (CNOM) ;
5. Location of practice;
6. Signature and stamp ;

7. Is the person to whom the certificate was issued mentioned. There are four types of medical-legal certificates:

1. Date of death ;

2. Time of Death ;

3. Is there a forensic obstacle?

4. Is there a requirement for immediate burial. A section to collect medical information:

Is the medical part of the certificate sealed?

A. Medical data:

▶ In Part I:

- Causes of death;
- The mechanism of death;
- The number of lines filled in this part (/4) ;
- Root cause;
- The immediate cause;
- Is the causal hierarchy respected?
- Is the time frame of the morbid conditions noted ;
- Is the writing legible?
- Are there any abbreviations.

▶ In Part II:

Other morbid or physiological conditions that may have contributed to the death.

B. Additional information:

- Presence of a pregnancy or childbirth within the last year ;
- Exact location of a possible accident ;
- Is it an accident at work ;
- Is the autopsy box checked?

3. ANALYSIS OF THE MEDICAL CERTIFICATE OF DEATH

The different sections of the CMD were studied and a quantitative and qualitative analysis of its content was made.

We have selected :

- A lack of data in the administrative section ;
- Two major groups of errors in causes of death: errors

major and minor errors ;

We conducted a review of the literature concerning the classification of errors in the writing of causes of death in CMDs and we tried to synthesize all these classifications.

Two groups of errors are essentially found. Major errors and

minor errors.

These major errors are errors that could distort the coding of the main cause of death by the National Institute of Public Health (INSP) according to the rules of the 10th revision of the International Classification of Diseases (ICD) or that could mislead on the exact circumstances and the medico-legal form of the death. There are six such errors:

- Only the mechanism of death is mentioned (no cause of death);
- The sequence of causes of death is incorrect;
- The cause of death is insufficient (thermal burns, road accident, polytrauma ...);
- Several causes of death are mentioned;
- Cause of death is unacceptable (clinical signs or symptoms,

physiological condition...);

- The box "presence of forensic obstacle" is unchecked.

Minor errors are less likely to bias the classification of the primary cause of death. There are five minor errors:

- The mechanism and cause of death are mentioned;
- The absence of the time interval between the onset of the disease and the occurrence of death ;
- The presence of inappropriate information (history of the victim, history of the disease ...) ;
- Illegible handwriting;
- The presence of abbreviations.

4. STATISTICAL ANALYSIS

Descriptive analyses were conducted using numbers and percentages for categorical variables and means and standard deviations for quantitative data. The bibliography analyzed incorporated the results of the PubMed/Medline bibliographic database search.

RESULTS

We conducted a prospective descriptive study, extended over a period of one year, including 74 CMD received at the Forensic Medicine Department of Habib Bourguiba Hospital in Sfax.

1. ADMINISTRATIVE COMPONENT

1.1. Demographic and sociological parameters concerning the deceased

We studied nine parameters concerning the demographic and sociological data of the deceased. All nine parameters were met in 8.1% of the CMDs. In more than half of the cases, more than six of the nine criteria were met. In 27.1% of the cases, there were less than four criteria mentioned (Table I). The average number of criteria met was 5.12.

Table I: Distribution of medical death certificates by number of socio-demographic criteria met

Total criteria met (out of nine)	**n (%)**
9	6 (8.1)
8	6 (8.1)
7	7 (9.5)
6	19 (25.7)
5	9 (12.2)
4	7 (9.5)
3	6 (8.1)
2	9 (12.2)
1	5 (6.8)
0	0 (0)
Total	**74 (100)**

The identity of the deceased (surname and first name) was the parameter that was present in all cases followed by age (90.5%), sex (77%), address (64.9%), national identity card number (52.7%), nationality (37.8%), marital status (33.8%) and while the place of death and occupation were most often absent, mentioned in 29.7% and 27% respectively (Table II)

Table II: Distribution of medical death certificates by socio-demographic data of the deceased

Criteria	Mentioned n (%)	Not mentioned n (%)	Total n (%)
First and last name	74 (100)	0 (0)	74 (100)
CIN number	39 (52.7)	35 (47.3)	74 (100)
Address	48 (64.9)	26 (35.1)	74 (100)
Age	67 (90.5)	7 (9.5)	74 (100)
Sex	57 (77)	17 (23)	74 (100)
Profession	20 (27)	54 (73)	74 (100)
Marital status	25 (33.8)	49 (66.2)	74 (100)
Nationality	28 (37.8)	46 (62.2)	74 (100)
Place of death	22 (29.7)	52 (70.3)	74 (100)

Age or date of birth was missing on 9.5% of CMDs. For children under 18 years of age, identity card number, occupation and marital status were left blank.

1.2. Data concerning the certifying physician

Of the seven criteria to be met in this section, 64.9% of certifying physicians met more than five criteria (Table III).

Table III: Distribution of medical death certificates according to the number of criteria met regarding the certifying physician

Total criteria met (out of seven)	n (%)
7	0 (0)
6	17 (23)
5	31 (41.9)
4	5 (6.8)
3	13 (17.6)
2	8 (10.8)
1	0 (0)
0	0 (0)
Total	74 (100)

On the CMD, the certifying doctor identified himself by his name, grade, speciality, CNOM registration number, place of practice and signature and/or stamp. The identification was satisfactory, mentioned in more than 90% of cases. On the other hand, in this part, the doctor only rarely mentioned to whom the certificate was issued (10.8%) (Table IV). The average number of criteria met was 5.5 ±1.3.

Table IV: Distribution of medical death certificates according to the percentage of completion of the criteria concerning the certifying physician

Criteria	Mentioned	Not mentioned	Total n (%)
	n (%)	n (%)	
Physician's name	74 (100)	0 (0)	74 (100)
Physician's specialty	62 (83.8)	12 (16.2)	74 (100)
Physician's rank	53 (71.6)	21 (28.4)	74 (100)
Registration number CNOM	16 (21.6)	58 (78.4)	74 (100)
Place of practice	54 (73)	20 (27)	74 (100)
Signature and stamp	72 (97.3)	2 (2.7)	74 (100)
The person to whom the			
certificate was issued	8 (10.8)	66 (89.2)	74 (100)
is it mentioned			

The speciality of the certifying doctor was specified in 83.8% of cases, mentioned on their stamp. More than half of the CMDs analysed were signed by specialist doctors, i.e. 21.6% of medical specialities and 47.3% of surgical specialities. In 79.7% of cases, the certifying doctors worked in hospitals, while 14.9% worked in the private sector. The certifying doctors were either general practitioners in public health (8.1%) or university hospital doctors (71.6%). University hospital doctors were represented by assistants (AHU) (14.9%), associate professors (32.4%) and professors (24.3%). Non-hospital academic physicians (23%) were represented by general practitioners and public health specialists as well as general practitioners and free-lance specialists.

1.3. Forensic data

The four boxes of the medico-legal data were filled in in more than three quarters of the CMDs, including the date of death and the OML box in more than 90% of the CMDs (Table V). In 26.6%, the OML section was either left blank (5.4%), or the doctor mentioned the absence of OML (4.05%), which was a major error because all the CMDs collected in our study were sent to the Forensic Medicine Department of Habib Bourguiba Hospital concerning corpses presenting a medico-legal obstacle to burial (Table VI).

Table V: Distribution of medical death certificates by completed forensic data

Criteria	Mentioned n(%)	Not mentioned n(%)
Date of death	74 (100)	0 (0)
Time of death	37 (50)	37 (50)
Heading for burial	64 (86.5)	10 (13.5)
OML section	70 (94.6)	4 (5.4)

Table VI: Distribution of medical death certificates by OML box data

Checked	Mentioned n (%)
Yes	67 (90.55)
No	3 (4.05)
No box checked	4 (5.4)
Total	74 (100)

In total, the administrative component was satisfactorily completed (more than 14 criteria mentioned) in about two thirds of the cases (52.8%). Two of the 74 CMDs had all 20 criteria met (Table VII). The minimum number of criteria met was five and the maximum was 20, for an average of 13 criteria.

Table VII: Distribution of medical death certificates according to the completion rate of the administrative part of the CMD (on 20 criteria)

Total criteria met (out of 20)	n (%)
20	2 (2.7)
19	0(0)
18	9(12.2)
17	1(1.4)
16	5 (6.8)
15	14 (18.9)
14	8 (10.8)
13	6 (8.1)
12	3 (4.1)
11	4 (5.4)
10	9 (12.2)
9	5 (6.8)
8	2 (2.7)

7	1 (1.4)
6	0 (0)
5	5 (6.8)
<=4	0 (0)
Total	74 (100)

2. MEDICAL ASPECTS

2.1. CMD Privacy

Although respecting confidentiality in CMD matters is a legal and ethical obligation, the doctor sealed the medical part in only 67.6% of cases.

2.2. Medical data

In this section, the certifying physician most often filled in only one line out of the four (36.5%). In 5.4% of cases, this section was left blank. (Table VIII).

Table VIII: Distribution of medical death certificates by number of lines completed

Number of completed line(s)	N (%)
0	4 (5.4)
1	27(36.5)
2	13 (17.6)
3	17 (23)
4	13 (17.6)
>=5	0 (0)
Total	74 (100)

The cause of death was mentioned in only 82.4% of the CMDs. In the remaining 16.6%, either the box was left blank, or "autopsy request" was mentioned, or only the mechanism of death was written. The initial cause was more frequently found than the immediate cause, i.e. 70.3% against 28.4%.

For the cause of death, the duration of the interval between the supposed start of the disease process and the date of death was mentioned in only 9.5% of cases. Part II of the medical section was rarely completed, in only 8.1% of cases (Table IX).

Table IX: Distribution of medical death certificates according to the completion rate of the different sections of the medical section

	Mentioned n (%)	Not mentioned n (%)
Cause of death	61 (82.4)	13 (17.6)
Initial cause	52 (70.3)	22 (29.7)
Immediate cause	21 (28.4)	53 (71.6)
Delay of morbid states	7 (9.5)	67 (90.5)
Part II	6 (8.1)	68 (91.9)

2.3. Additional information

This section was left blank in 71.6% of cases. On the other hand, in 76.3% of the cases, the certifying doctors answered the question "has an autopsy been or will be performed".

3. ANALYSIS OF THE QUALITY OF WRITING

In our study, all CMDs contained at least one major and/or one minor error.

3.1. The major errors

In 17.6% of the CMDs, there were no major errors. In the remaining CMDs, there was only one major error (33.8%). No CMD contained more than four major errors (Table X).

Table X: Distribution of the number of major errors on the medical certificate of death

Number of major errors	N (%)
Without major error	13 (17.6)
A major mistake	25 (33.8)
Two major mistakes	16 (21.6)
Three major mistakes	10 (13.5)
Four major mistakes	10 (13.5)
Five or more major errors	0 (0)
Total	74 (100)

There were six major error types:

- Only the mechanism of death was mentioned

This error was encountered in 59.5% of CMDs. It was the most frequent major error. The mechanisms of death encountered were: cardiorespiratory arrest, multivisceral failure and shock.

- The sequence of causes of death was incorrect

This type of error was found in 40.5% of CMDs. Most certifying physicians put the initial cause on line a of the medical part until the immediate cause that led to death on the last line. Others wrote several causes of death on the same line.

- The cause of death was insufficient This error was found in 41.9% of CMDs.
- Several causes of death were mentioned

This major error was not found in any CMD.

- The cause of death was unacceptable

This error was found in 27% of CMDs. Most often, the certifying physicians used terms such as elderly subject to determine the cause of death or, sometimes, they recorded symptoms or a clinical sign.

- The box "presence of forensic obstacle" was unchecked

Although all the CMDs collected in our study had an impediment to burial, all 90.5% of the certifying physicians indicated the presence of a medico-legal impediment by checking "yes" under "medico-legal impediment to burial". In the remaining cases, the physician checked "no" to

The patient either did not answer "OML at burial" or did not answer this item, leaving the two boxes blank. OML was not mentioned most often in children or when the cause of death was not mentioned and sometimes even in sudden death.

In total, the most frequent major error was the mention of the mechanism of death alone without the cause of death (59.5%), followed by insufficient cause of death (41.9%), followed by the incorrect sequencing of causes of death (40.5%) and the box "presence of OML" not checked (9.5%) (Table XI).

Table XI: Distribution of different types of major errors in medical death certificates

Type of major error	N (%)
Only the death mechanism is mentioned	44 (59.5)
The cause of death sequence is incorrect	30 (40.5)
Cause of death is insufficient	31 (41.9)
Several causes of death are mentioned	0 (0)
Cause of death is unacceptable	20 (27)
The box "presence of OML" is not checked	7 (9.5)

3.2. Minor errors

All CMDs contained at least one minor error. No CMD contained more than four minor errors (Table XII).

Table XII: Distribution of the number of minor errors on the medical certificate of death

Number of minor errors	N (%)
No minor errors	0 (0)
A minor error	8 (10.8)
Two minor errors	16 (21.6)
Three minor errors	33 (44.6)
Four minor errors	17 (23)
Five minor errors	0 (0)
Total	74 (100)

There were five types of minor errors:

- Lack of time interval between the onset of the disease and the occurrence of death

This error was found in three quarters of the CMDs (29.7%). In these cases, the time interval column was left blank.

- Mechanism and cause(s) of death mentioned This error was found in 66.2% of CMDs. The mechanisms of death followed by the cause of death most frequently encountered were cardiorespiratory arrest, multivisceral failure, respiratory distress and shock. They were indicated, generally on line a, as the immediate cause of death followed by the cause of death.

- Inappropriate informationThis error was found in 43.2% of CMDs. The inappropriate information found was the history of the deceased and the history of the disease.

- Illegible handwriting The certifying physician's handwriting was found to be illegible in 21.6% of cases.

- Presence of abbreviation(s) This error was found in 87.8% of CMDs. It was the most frequently observed minor error among all the errors. Although some abbreviations were relatively clear (MVA: motor vehicle accident, CT: head injury, APO: acute pulmonary oedema), others were more difficult to interpret (VD: multivessel failure).

In **total,** among the minor errors, the presence of abbreviations was by far the most frequent error (in 87.8% of cases). Illegible handwriting was the least frequent error. (Table XIII).

Table XIII: Distribution of different types of minor errors in medical death certificates

Type of minor error	N (%)
The absence of a time interval between the onset of the disease and the occurrence of death	22 (29.7)
Mechanism and cause of death mentioned	49 (66.2)
The presence of inappropriate information	32 (43.2)
An illegible handwriting	16 (21.6)
Presence of abbreviations	65 (87.8)

DISCUSSION

Death necessarily involves the intervention of a doctor. It should be recalled that death was defined by the decision of the Minister of Public Health on 16 October 1998 as follows "Either the irreversible cessation of cardiorespiratory function; or the irreversible cessation of all encephalic functions. This decision specifies that only a medical doctor is authorized to declare the occurrence of death. In order to establish the declaration of death, the civil registrar must have in his possession a medical certificate attesting to the death [10]. We studied 74 CMDs. The quality of writing was unsatisfactory since only 17.6% of the CMDs were free of errors. Although the results are interesting, the small sample size was the weak point of this study.

1. THE MEDICAL CERTIFICATE OF DEATH: RULES FOR DRAFTING AND ISSUING

1.1. The certifying physician

Any doctor called upon to record a death must draw up a certificate. In Tunisia, unlike in France, this task is reserved for medical doctors who have obtained their medical degree and are registered with the Order of Physicians. In France, even a doctor who has not obtained his or her medical degree and who is replacing a private practitioner, on the sole condition that this replacement is carried out within a strict regulatory framework and subject to the prior information of the Regional Council of the Order of the department concerned, may draw up a CMD. Therefore, residents who have not obtained their medical degree and interns are not allowed to sign the CMD [9,10]. However, if this task is entrusted to an intern in a hospital, it is with the authorisation and under the responsibility of the department head. On the other hand, in Anglo-Saxon countries such as Australia, Canada, New Zealand and South Africa, the CMD can be completed and signed not only by a physician but also by a coroner. The coroner is a public official who is responsible for investigating the circumstances of a death involving an OML. The role of the coroner is to determine the causes and circumstances of death while investigating whether the death could have been prevented, to protect the living by making recommendations to prevent similar deaths, and to inform the public about the probable medical causes and circumstances of death [11].

If the doctor does not have official pre-printed certificates, the CMD may, exceptionally, be written on plain paper: it then simply specifies the presumed time and date of death, the commune where the death occurred, as well as the communicated identity of the victim if known [9].

The CMD must not be confused with the descriptive certificate (of injuries) often requested by the police in the event of a death on the public highway. The latter document, which must not mention the cause of death, can only be issued on the written request of a judicial police officer, the National Guard or the public prosecutor. The CMD must not be assimilated to a burial permit, an administrative document that will only be produced at a later stage by a civil registrar, after reception of the CMD and drafting of the death certificate [6, 7, 12].

1.2. PDC Model

Decree No. 99-1043 of 17 May 1999, published in the Journal Officiel de la République Tunisienne No. 43 of 28 May 1999 [4], established the model for the medical death certificate and the information it must contain. The latter conforms to the international model that has been established and recommended since 1948 by the World Health Organization to all member states.

Several ministerial circulars have subsequently reinforced and recalled the mandatory nature of the use of this model for the public and private sectors. This form is available from the official printers of the Republic of Tunisia [5]. The public health structures are responsible for supplying the various services with these certificates. The council of the order makes them available to private doctors. The death certificate is also an administrative document drawn up by the civil registrar of the presumed place of death, as stipulated in article 44 of the law relating to civil status [13]: "the death certificate will be drawn up by the civil registrar of the district where the death occurred, on the declaration of a relative of the deceased or on that of a person who has the most accurate and complete information on his or her civil status that is possible. No burial shall be made without an authorization, on free paper and without charge, from the civil registrar. The law punishes with imprisonment of up to 6 months, any person who causes a deceased person to be buried without prior authorization from the registrar. The death certificate allows the inheritance procedures to begin and allows the payment of capital (life insurance, loan repayments, etc.) [13-15]. The administrative section must be filled in, printed in duplicate and signed by the certifying doctor [12]. The deadline for declaring a death at home is three days [13]. In the case of a death occurring in a hospital or in a hospital unit, the declaration must be made within 24 hours by the person in charge of the establishment in order to inform the civil registrar [13,16].

Currently in France, the medical aspect differs according to the age of the death. In fact, a green certificate is available to doctors for the deaths of children born alive and who died between birth and the 27th day of life, as long as the gestational age is 22 weeks of amenorrhea and/or the child's weight at birth is more than 500 g (with the exception of stillbirths), and a blue certificate is available for deaths from 28 days of life [12]. In Tunisia, there is no specific CMD for newborns and the model used is that of adults with the possibility, in the causes of death section, of including causes related to a maternal pathology, such as premature rupture of the membranes, infection, etc. However, a project to set up a model of neonatal death certificate is underway at the INSP [12].

1.3. Composition of the CMD

According to the model of the medical certificate of death established by decree n°99-1043 of 17 May 1999 in the Official Gazette of the Tunisian Republic n°43 of 28 May 1999 [2], this certificate has a front and a back (Annex 2).

The RECTO: It contains a number of data of different order

spread over two distinct parts:

The upper part: this is the administrative part, it is nominative and relates to the civil status, it must be signed by the doctor who must also affix his stamp. This part is itself divided into three sections:

Demographic and sociological parameters concerning the deceased:

Surname and first name(s), National Identity Card number, address, age, sex, occupation, marital status, nationality and place of death.

Data concerning the certifying physician :

The name, specialty, grade, registration number with the National Council of the Order of Physicians (CNOM), place of practice, signature and stamp of the physician and the person to whom the certificate was issued.

Forensic data:

On the date and time of death. It also makes it possible to specify the presence or not of a medico-legal obstacle as well as the necessity or not of immediate burial.

* The forensic obstacle must be ticked when the death occurs unexpectedly and unexplained or in the case of a violent death (accidental, tortious, suicidal or criminal death) or suspicious (unknown cause). The body will then be placed at the disposal of the justice, an investigation is always opened and a forensic autopsy is often requested. The notions of suspicious or violent death have been referred to in the following regulations:

- Article 48 of law n° 57-3 of 1 August 1957 regulating civil status [13], specifies that: "When there are signs or indications of violent death or other circumstances that give reason to suspect it, burial may only be carried out after a police officer, assisted by a Medical Doctor, has drawn up a report on the state of the corpse and the circumstances relating to it, as well as the information he has been able to gather on the first name, surname, age, profession, place of birth and domicile of the deceased."

- Article n°28 of decree N°81-1634 of 30 November 1981 concerning the general internal regulations of hospitals, institutes and specialised centres under the Ministry of Public Health [17] specifies that: "in the event of signs or indications of violent or suspicious death of a hospitalised patient, the Director, informed by the Head of Department, shall immediately notify the judicial authority, in accordance with the legislation in force".

- Paragraph 2 of article n° 7 of decree n° 97-1326 of July 7, 1997 relating to the modalities of preparation of graves and fixing the rules of burial and exhumation of mortal remains or corpses [14] stipulates that "in case of death resulting from violence, accident or other doubtful circumstances, burial can only be authorized in accordance with the provisions of article 48 of the law relating to the civil status".

* The obligation of immediate burial concerns certain contagious, epidemic or infectious diseases. According to the decree n° 97- 1326 of July 7, 1997, relating to the modalities of preparation of the graves and fixing the rules of burial and exhumation of mortal remains or corpses[14], the diseases concerned are: cholera, rabies, AIDS, viral hepatitis except confirmed hepatitis A and viral hemorrhagic fevers.

The lower part: this is the medical part. It is anonymous and must be sealed by the physician immediately after it is written in order to preserve the confidentiality of the causes of death. It will only be opened at the National Institute of Public Health (INSP) by the public health physician in charge of the entry and coding of the medical causes of death.

This part has two sections:

Causes of death: these **are** divided into two sections:

i. Part I: Leading causes of death: These are all the diseases, morbid conditions or injuries that led to or contributed to the death and the circumstances of the accident or violence that led to these injuries and not the mechanism of death (cardio-respiratory arrest, dehydration, heart failure, respiratory failure). This section has four lines that allow the physician to describe the causal sequence of illnesses that led directly to death, from the last or immediate cause corresponding to the condition or morbid state directly responsible for death, reported on "line a", to the initial or terminal cause that inaugurated the sequence of events between normal health and death, reported on the last line of this part I. This initial cause of death is defined by WHO as:

- The disease or trauma that triggered the disease process leading directly to death or ;
- The circumstances of the accident or violence that led to the fatal injury.

The initial cause of death is therefore the cause that must be acted upon to prevent death. It is this cause that will be used primarily to present medical mortality statistics.

The length of the interval between the presumed onset of the disease process and the date of death must be indicated for each condition listed on the certificate.

ii. Part II: where the physician will record other morbid or physiological conditions that adversely affected the course of the disease process, and thus contributed to the fatal outcome, but were not related to the disease or morbid condition that directly caused the death. These are the so-called associated causes.

Additional information

Including a possible link to a pregnancy or childbirth within the last year, the exact location of a possible accident, the place of death and whether a medical autopsy has been or will be performed.

THE BACK PAGE: it contains information on the regulations concerning the completion of the administrative section and examples of how to complete the medical section.

2. FILLING IN THE DIFFERENT SECTIONS OF THE CMD

2.1. Administrative component

2.1.1. Socio-demographic data on the deceased

In our study, the sociodemographic data were completely filled in, i.e. nine criteria, in only 8.1% of the FDCs. In more than half of the CMDs, more than six criteria were met. Burger et al [4] noted that socio-demographic data such as age, marital status and origin were mentioned in more than 2/3 of the FDCs. El Nour et al [18] found that they were filled in 92.8% of the cases. Haque et al [19] found that in 92% of the FDCs, there were errors or missing data in these socio-demographic data. Another study [20] found a lot of errors in recording the place of residence of the deceased on the CMD. Sibai et al [21] noted that the deceased's occupation and age were most often missing from the CMD, in 95% and 78% respectively.

When writing the CMD, these socio-demographic parameters may in some cases pose a problem for the doctor making the finding:

- when the identity of the deceased is unknown, the doctor can leave it under X, which

involves checking the "forensic obstacle" box for identification.

- If death occurred in an ambulance en route to the hospital, the name of the hospital should be entered as the place of death. If the death occurred on a sea or air conveyance, it is recommended that the name of the ship (at sea) or the flight number be recorded [22].

2.1.2. Data concerning the certifying physician

Concerning the data on the certifying physician, Sibai et al [21] noted that about half of the certificates did not contain a signature of the certifying physician. In the study by El Nour et al [18], the certifying physician's signature and stamp were absent in 18% of CMDs, whereas in our study they were absent in 2.7% of cases. The physician's signature was often absent at the extreme ages of life and more often in women[21].

2.1.3. Forensic data

Regarding the date and time of death, attention must be paid to the day, month and year of death. The doctor may be faced with a delicate situation when he does not know the date and time of death. In this case, he can put either the date and time of discovery of the corpse (by expressly stating it), or the estimated date and time of death (by mentioning for example "appearing to be from"), referring to his thanatological knowledge [23]. In the case of a death with an OML, this information will be confirmed later by the forensic expert [11]. As for the heading "entombment", it concerns contagious or epidemic diseases and sometimes, in certain countries such as France, the poor condition of the body, including in particular the more or less advanced state of putrefaction. If the death is due to a transmissible disease, it must be declared in writing to the health authority, which is represented by a doctor or a biologist under the Ministry of Public Health, specially appointed to carry out this mission. In our Tunisian model, the diseases that must be reported immediately are contagious, epidemic or infectious diseases such as cholera, rabies, AIDS, viral hepatitis except hepatitis A and viral hemorrhagic fevers [2]. The list of contagious diseases justifying burial has been modified in France (since 1998) to include the plague, all HIV infections and no longer AIDS, and in case of absence of burial within six days after death. However, hepatitis A is no longer mentioned [24]. Unlike the Tunisian CMD, the French CMD includes other headings than OML or burial, such as cremation, conservation care, transport of the body and a heading for "sampling in order to search for the cause of death". This is the medical autopsy, also called scientific autopsy. It is indicated whenever the cause of death is unknown and there is no OML. Scientific autopsies are performed outside the judicial framework in order to obtain a diagnosis on the cause of death. They are carried out by anatomopathologists without the presence of the authorities or the sealing of samples. It is carried out at the request of doctors (sometimes requested in writing by the family) and can take place if the deceased person did not object during his or her lifetime. This refusal can be expressed by any means, in particular by registration in an automated register, this choice being revocable at any time. This register of refusals must be consulted beforehand. In the absence of knowledge of the wishes of the deceased, the doctor must obtain the consent of the family according to the same procedures as those for obtaining consent for the removal of organs from the deceased for scientific or therapeutic purposes.

2.2. Medical component

2.2.1. CMD Privacy

The lower part contains confidential medical information, which justifies the sealing of this document when it is handed over to the family. The confidentiality of the data reproduced on the medical section of the death certificate is a legal obligation, as stipulated in article 254 of the Tunisian Criminal Code (CPT): "Doctors, surgeons and other health workers, pharmacists, midwives and all other persons who, by virtue of their status or profession, are entrusted with secrets, will have revealed these secrets, except in cases where the law obliges or authorizes them to act as informers."The Code of Medical Ethics (CDM) states that "professional secrecy is imposed on all doctors, except in cases of derogation established by law" and that "the doctor must ensure that the persons who assist him in his work are informed of their obligations in terms of professional secrecy and comply with them". In spite of this, we noted in our study that in 32.4% of cases the confidential part was not sealed. Different results were observed in the study carried out in the forensic medicine department of the Garches University Hospital in France. Indeed, 75% of the death certificates studied were not sealed. The author underlines this fact and probably attributes it to oversights, or to a reluctance of the doctors to lick the sticky part of the certificate (moreover the doctors questioned in this study would like a sticky certificate). Sometimes, the certificate can be old and difficult to stick. However, it is necessary to recall that in Tunisia as elsewhere, leaving the medical part of the death certificate unsealed, engages the responsibility of the physician, and exposes him to penal and ordinal sanctions related to the disclosure of information covered by medical secrecy [25-26].

2.2.2. **Filling in the medical data**

The CMD is a document on which the physician reports various information on the circumstances of the death and the cause of its occurrence. This document is the main source for relevant national mortality statistics [27]. The information on the CMD must be accurate and as complete as possible in order to allow the classification of causes of death, which is the basic tool for comparing death statistics between different regions of the country and between countries, in order to make funding decisions for research and development and to identify health priorities. A poorly written, incomplete CMD can lead to inaccurate health statistics, inaccurate calculations of disease prevalence, and unequal distribution of health resources and budgets across regions.The medical section of the CMD consists of two separate parts and a series of additional information to be filled in according to the context.

In **Part I**, which corresponds to the causal chain of diseases that led directly to death:

Only one cause of death is listed on each line.

Line a must be filled in. If the cause on line a is the consequence of another disease state, it must be marked on the next line b and so on until the entire causal chain is completed [22]. The word "chain" refers to a sequence of two or more disease states listed in Part I on successive lines, each of which can be considered a plausible cause of the one listed in the previous line. In some circumstances, the immediate cause is itself the initial cause of death. Lines should not be skipped. Additional lines can be added as needed [22].

The initial cause should always be reported on the last line of this **Part I** without being required to complete all four lines. If the certifying physician does not know the cause of death, it should be reported as unknown, undetermined, probable, or unspecified so that it is clear that the cause has not been carelessly omitted. When the distinction between immediate and initial cause is not respected, discrepancies in interpretation may arise [22]. In all cases, causes of death that are not causally related should not be listed on successive lines in Part I [28].For each condition listed on the certificate, the length of the interval between the presumed onset of the disease process and the date of death should be indicated, with the time interval from the immediate cause listed in the first line to the time interval of the initial cause increasing [28]. The terms "not known", "approximate", minutes, hours or days may be used. This box should not be left blank [22].The mechanism of death such as respiratory arrest, cardiac arrest, asystole, cardiorespiratory arrest, ventricular fibrillation, renal failure, shock and sepsis should not be included as a cause of death but if noted it should always be followed by the cause(s) of death, e.g. cardiac arrest due to coronary atherosclerosis or cardiac arrest due to blunt trauma to the chest [19 The etiology of visceral failure such as congestive heart failure, liver failure, renal failure, or respiratory failure should be included on the CMD, e.g., renal failure due to type 1 diabetes.When death occurred following surgical treatment, the reason for the treatment should be included as well as the type of surgery performed [29]. It is also important to specify the etiology of peritonitis, e.g., is it complicated appendicitis, perforated peptic ulcer, or some other etiology. In the case of trauma, the location of the trauma that caused the death should be indicated and the circumstances or cause of the trauma should be specified. In the case of intoxication or overdose, the name of the product, drug or substance involved must be specified. If it is unknown to the certifying physician, it is also advisable to mention it. El Nour et al [18] found that the cause of death was completed in 98.5% of CMDs. These results are consistent with those found in our study, since part I was completed in 95% of CMDs, but the cause of death was mentioned in only 83.3%, because instead of mentioning the cause of death, the certifying physician entered the mechanism of death alone, or put "request for forensic autopsy" or "body disposal", or mentioned a symptom such as "constipation", or described signs found during the pre- or post-mortem clinical examination, such as "ecchymosis Although part II was completed in 100% of CMDs in Agarwal's study [30], in most studies it is rarely completed by certifying physicians. Burger et al [13] reported 8.5% use of this part. El Nour et al [18] found this section completed in 3% of CMDs. In our study, this section was completed in only 10.8% of the CMDs, which is a very low rate and shows that certifying physicians focus essentially on the cause of death without paying attention to the importance of this section and its interest in the classification of diseases that may be involved in the death or constitute a risk factor for the occurrence of death.

3. EDITING ERRORS

Different classifications have been reported in the literature: We tried to synthesize and adapt all these classifications (which were not very different) to finally apply our classification mentioned in the methods chapter. In a study carried out in Tunisia [31,32], the assessment of the quality of the declaration of causes of death on the certificates showed that only 89.7% of the certificates received by the INSP in 2009 contained sufficiently clear indications on the morbid condition that led to death. This rate of notification of causes of death had improved significantly over the years. Indeed, it was 89.3% in 2006, 86.2% in 2003 and 80% in 2001. In another Tunisian study [33], the cause of death was mentioned in only 44.1% of all deaths. The percentage of correctly written CMDs with no major or minor errors varied greatly according to the studies, ranging from 1% in Pakistan
[19] to 80% in Taiwan [34].

This difference between the studies was explained by several reasons:

- The WDC model itself: each country has adapted the WHO model by simplifying it or adding more boxes to be filled in.

- Training of the certifying physician: in England, regular training of physicians likely to write a CMD has made it possible to improve the percentage of error-free certificates (up to 71%) [7].

- The lack of information on the scope of the CMD and the relevance of this certificate in the realization of statistics and in the implementation of prevention campaigns.

- Lack of experience in writing CMDs, fatigue, lack of time and lack of knowledge of the deceased's medical history [35].

The classification adopted in the majority of studies was twofold

groups of errors: major and minor errors.

3.1. The major errors

Major errors could lead to miscoding of the primary cause of death.

These errors were:

Only the mechanism of death was mentioned (absence of cause of death): This error accounted for 7% of major errors in the study by Lu et al [3]. In 13.5% of CMDs in South Africa, the mechanism of death was mentioned as the only cause of death or was followed by a cause of death but no link was found between the mechanism and that cause [4]. The mechanism of death was the most frequent type of error in the English study with 20% of CMDs [7], and the Greek study with 34.5% of CMDs [4]. This type of error accounted for 62% of CMDs in the Pakistani study [19], 47% in the Sudanese study [18] and only 9.9% and 5.7% of CMDs in the Canadian and Taiwanese studies respectively (Table XIV) [34,36]. In our study, the mechanism of death alone, not followed by the cause of death, was found in 59.5% of DCMs.

- The sequence of causes of death was incorrect; the sequence of causes of death must be clear and complete in order to convey the information necessary to understand the sequence of events leading to death. CMDs with this type of error contained little information for epidemiological data [5]. If, after careful consideration, the certifying physician was unable to determine a causal sequence for the occurrence of death, the OML box should be checked. This error may be explained by the lack of training on how to record the cause of death, immediate cause in the first line, then intermediate causes and finally the initial cause in the last line of the causal sequence [18]. Other difficulties have also been reported by certifying physicians in determining the sequence of medical causes in elderly persons with multiple pathologies [37].

- The cause of death was insufficient: The cause of death was mentioned but lacked precision or was absent such as a tumour without specifying its malignancy or benignity, a cancer without specifying the primary site, a stroke without specifying the type (haemorrhagic or ischemic), digestive haemorrhage without specifying the site, a road accident without specifying the circumstances of occurrence (pedestrian, driver, passenger, motorcyclist...). This error could be explained on the one hand by the duration of the illness that contributed to the death. If a person dies after a long, well-known illness, the cause of death in the CMD is complete and precise. Whereas the cause of death is less precise or insufficient when the disease was recently diagnosed [19].

On the other hand, in the case of deaths occurring in hospital or during an on-call period, the certifying physician, not being the attending physician, might lack the time or the motivation to consult the medical record [35]. Ideally, the certifying physician could be contacted for further information. In France, a study carried out among 14 general practitioners [38] reminded us that the certification of deaths is an act that is not very frequent, unless they work in a home hospitalization network for palliative care. None of the doctors interviewed in this study recalled having received university training in death certification.

Nevertheless, all considered this act to be part of their duties. On the other hand, many refuted the idea of moving without delay, leaving their consultations, to go to the body. Very few examined the deceased after undressing, even less so when the family or the nursing staff prepared him for burial. All these practices compromised the quality of death certification [37].

- Several causes of death were mentioned: On the CMD, the certifying physician should mention only one causal chain of death, but in practice, this is difficult because the deceased had several concomitant diseases or traumas that could have led to death [36]. This error was not found in any CMDs in our study, compared with 2.3% and 4% in the Taiwanese studies [3, 34].

- The cause of death was unacceptable: On the CMD of elderly or newborns there should be a clear and complete causal chain if possible. Terms such as senescence, infirmity, old age, advanced age, asthenia, prematurity or unnatural death have little value for public health or medical research, as do clinical signs and symptoms. Burger et al [4] found this error in 14.8% of CMDs and Armour et al [8] in only 3.6%. In our study, it was 27%.
- The box "presence of forensic obstacle" was unchecked:

This major error is quite frequent in our study, estimated at 9.5%: 5.4% left this box blank instead of checking OML and 4.05% mentioned the absence of OML.

With regard to the medico-legal obstacle, the certifying physician must indicate the presence of an OML at burial in a number of cases. However, it is true that the certifying physician lacks information on the causes that may constitute an OML [13]. When faced with a death, the certifying physician may have two options:

In case of natural death or death that does not pose a forensic problem:
Natural death is the expected death resulting from the evolution of a pathological condition of the individual or the end of his or her aging process. In other words, it is the consequence of a known pathological process (the deceased was medically monitored and his or her death does not come as a great surprise) or unknown, detectable or undetectable, not involving any directly responsible external third party. The formalities prescribed by the Civil Registry are then very simple in order to proceed with the burial. The declaration of death in the case of death by natural causes is a legal and ethical obligation of the doctor. In fact, the president of the commune must only issue the burial permit on production of a death certificate issued by the doctor [39]. This type of situation is frequently encountered in hospitals. In private practice, the doctor treating the deceased is often in the best position to attest the naturalness of the death, as he recognises the pathological past of his patient [9].

Generally speaking, caution is the rule. The absence of external traumatic signs in no way eliminates internal trauma or toxic death (whose criminal etiology is not excluded). Furthermore, it should be remembered that the presence of external traumatic signs can be seen in some natural deaths, such as a fainting spell followed by a fall.

In the event of a death that poses a forensic problem :
This situation includes cases of violent, sudden, suspicious death or death of unknown cause. These deaths pose a medico-legal obstacle to burial and the doctor, who has a decisive medico-social role here as an auxiliary of justice, must not hesitate either to simply mention that the death is of unknown cause or that it poses a medico-legal problem. In this case a judicial inquiry is always opened and a forensic autopsy is often requested by the judicial authorities.

In general, the physician should check the OML box in these three cases:
- **Violent death:** Violent death includes death resulting from the use of force or from the intervention of a sudden and brutal external cause and raises the hypothesis of a possible crime or offence. Violent death has been classified into three categories: accidents, suicides and homicides.

- Accidents (on the public highway, at work and in the home): involuntary acts where death is directly related to an accidental trauma and the causal link is often obvious. When the facts are of a tortious nature, such as a fatal road accident with the possibility of a third party being responsible, it is necessary to tick off the medico-legal obstacle. In France, the practice of autopsy after an accident is not the rule: this is not the case in our country, in Germany and in Sweden where the use of autopsy in such circumstances is more systematic [9].
- Suicides: actions to voluntarily cause one's own death. The suicidal nature of the death can only be established after careful police and forensic investigations including an autopsy. The doctor who signs the CMD must be aware that it is not his responsibility to decide on the

suicidal cause of death, but that it is up to the courts (mainly the public prosecutor) to do so. In the case of suicide at home, the doctor's mission is to confirm the death, to try to comfort the family and friends, but also to explain the reason for the OML at the burial and its consequences. To establish, as the relatives of the deceased sometimes insist, a certificate attesting that the death is of natural cause when it is apparently a suicide, constitutes a serious fault exposing the doctor to both disciplinary and legal proceedings [9].

- Homicide: the voluntary or involuntary action of a third party caused the death. Criminal action is very likely, but the crime can also be hidden under the most diverse masks: accident, suicide and possibly natural death. A suspected or obvious criminal death therefore requires that the OML be checked.

- **Suspicious death:** any death which, at first sight, cannot be clearly explained, or which may involve a third party, or which occurs in unusual circumstances, or which may be the result of an offence, is suspicious in the eyes of the law. The basis of suspicious death is doubt: this suspicion refers to the personality of the deceased (criminal, delinquent, public figure, risky profession), to the circumstances of the occurrence of the death (during a medical or paramedical procedure, a quarrel, an offence) or of the discovery of the body (corpse found in an isolated vacant lot), the statements made by the family, neighbours or even circulating public rumour, lesions compatible with traces of violence found on the body of the deceased, implausibilities when the body was discovered (incoherent signs of death such as broken rigor mortis or paradoxical lividity). In all cases of suspicious death, the duty is to report the OML.

- **Sudden death:** is defined as a natural death, which occurs unexpectedly in a subject in apparent good health within a short period of time after the appearance of any symptoms, i.e. after a brief agony. The characteristics of sudden death make it a highly suspicious death in the eyes of all, which often explains why it is explored in a medico-legal context. Indeed, a forensic expertise is requested by the justice in order to specify the natural or not character of this death. A death that is not expected remains unnatural until there is forensic evidence to the contrary and the doctor must tick the OML box on the CMD. In summary, in the event of any forensic obstacle, the police inform the public prosecutor, and the body is then placed at the disposal of justice. The public prosecutor (sometimes a judicial police officer or the investigating judge if an investigation has been opened) decides whether or not to carry out an external examination of the body. The decision whether or not to carry out an autopsy rests with the prosecutor in the light of the investigators' initial findings. The prosecutor may "remove the obstacle" and authorise burial. The relatives of the deceased may neither demand nor oppose a judicial autopsy. In the case of a forensic autopsy, the report cannot be given directly to the treating physician or the family by the forensic physician. To obtain the results of post-mortem examinations, relatives or their lawyers must apply directly to the magistrate in charge of the death. It is the magistrate who will decide what to communicate to the parties [24,40].

Table XIV: Types of major errors by study

	Uniquement le mécanisme de décès mentionné (%)	Enchainement incorrect des causes de décès (%)	Cause de décès insuffisante ou non spécifique (%)	Plusieurs causes de décès mentionnées (%)	Cause de décès inacceptable (%)	Case OML non cochée (%)
Lu et al. [4]	7	9	19	4		
Burger et al. [5]	13,5	28,7		15,3	14,8	
Katsakiori et al. [6]	34,5	6,8	4,5	14,8		
Kathryn et al. [7]	15,8	15,8			7,5	
Slater et al. [8]	20%	6	6			
Armour et al. [9]	5,2	7,3	15,8		3,6	
Jordan et al. [40]	9,9	22,3		17,1		
Patel et al. [42]		55		5		
Cheng et al. [44]	5,7	3,6	8,3	2,3		

3.2. Minor errors

Minor errors were found both in our study, in the order of 100%, and in other studies such as the South African study which found 86.1% minor errors (Table XV) [4]. We classified the minor errors into five groups:

- The absence of the time interval between the onset of the disease and the

Most certifying doctors paid little attention to this section because of the lack of information on the interest of filling in this part. Indeed, this time interval made it possible to know the sequence of events and facilitated the work of nosologists faced with a poorly written CMD by allowing them to follow and interpret the sequence of events that led to death and to determine the initial cause [4,6,28]. It was the most frequently encountered minor error in the different studies, unlike in our study, where it was 29.7%, and 92.5% [41], 81.5% [4], 69.2% [6], 63% [30] and 35.9% [36] in
other studies.

- Both the mechanism and cause of death are mentioned:

Not only was the mechanism of death mentioned, but also the specific cause of death. This was an error, but less serious than listing only the mechanism of death as the cause of death. This error was found in 66.2% of our study, in 45.9% of the Canadian study by Myers et al [6] and in 80% of the Indian study by Patel et al [41].

- Presence of inappropriate information (history of the victim, history of the disease, etc.): Information of no interest in the classification of causes of death was found in the medical part of the CMD. This type of error was encountered in 43.2% of the certificates in our study, 13% in the study by Myers et al [6] and 6.1% in the study by Sibai et al [21]. Inappropriate information was reported such as the history of the deceased or the history of the disease. The history should normally be written in part II of the associated causes if it adversely affected the course of the disease process, and thus contributed to the fatal outcome, but was not related to the disease or condition that directly caused the death. The history of the disease has sometimes been written in paragraph form.

- Illegible handwriting:

Illegible handwriting was a very subjective finding, either because the handwriting was totally illegible or because it was very difficult to read. It could also be explained by the certifying physicians' lack of awareness of the importance of the information on the CMD and the consequences of illegible handwriting on the classification of causes of death and the resulting errors. Burger et al [4] found this type of error in 2.5% of CMDs, whereas Patel et al [41] found it in 15% of CMDs. In our study, it was 21.6%.

- The presence of abbreviations :

This type of error has been encountered in several studies, and varies from 9.8% [18] to 32.5% [41]. In our study, it was 87.8%. The most frequently found abbreviations were MVA for Motor Vehicle Accident, RCA for Cardiopulmonary Arrest and APO for Acute Pulmonary Oedema. There were also other abbreviations such as VMD for Multivessel Failure, ARDS for Acute Respiratory Distress Syndrome, CT for Traumatic Brain Injury, TT for Traumatic Chest Injury ... The certifying physician could not, in some situations, decode the abbreviation. Even worse, he could misinterpret it. For example, BAV which could mean Auriculo-Ventricular Block or Decreased Visual Acuity, IVC which could mean either Inter-Ventricular Communication or Intravenous Catheter, HCM for Hypertrophic Cardiomyopathy or Hypertensive Cardiomyopathy, DA for Artificial Delivery or Aortic Dissection, MI for Mitral Insufficiency or Intramuscular Injection, CRI for Chronic Renal Failure or Chronic Respiratory Failure, CCP for Chronic Constrictive Pericarditis or Chronic Calcifying Pancreatitis, AP for Acute Pancreatitis or Acute Prostatitis In summary, all these minor errors could be due to inexperience, lack of time, fatigue or a certain degree of carelessness on the part of the certifying physician [35,42].

Table XV: Percentage of different types of minor errors in the literature

	Absence d'intervalle de temps entre l'apparition de la maladie et la survenue du décès %	Mécanisme et cause de décès mentionnés %	Informations non appropriées %	Ecriture illisible %	Présence d'abréviations %
Burger et al. [5]	81,5		13	2,5	23,7
Kathryn et al. [7]	69,2	45,9			19,9
Jordan et al. [40]	35,9		6,1		9,8
Patel et al. [42]	92,5	80		15	32,5

4. RECOMMENDATIONS

Certain measures can be taken to reduce the frequency of errors in the writing of the cause of death, mainly concerning training, final CMDs and the certifying physician.

4.1. Concerning the training of certifying doctors

Recalling that in our medical training, the student receives only one hour of theoretical teaching on the CMD and this in the course "diagnosis and legislation of death" in the framework of the certificate of Legal Medicine taught in DCEM 3. This seems very little given the importance of this document. In all the articles published recently, doctors, whatever their speciality, deplore insufficient training [19, 38, 43, 44].

Initial training should explain the epidemiological importance of death certification, so that future physicians become aware of the importance of performing this procedure, given that the majority lack information on the value of PDCs. In a 2007 study of family physicians in Canada, very few physicians were aware of the usefulness of CMDs, most knew that they were used for mortality statistics but were unaware of their importance in epidemiological statistics and the planning and evaluation of health care programs [38,44].

However, while all physicians agree that certifying death is part of their job, they are not sure how to do it. Thus, explaining to all future doctors that visiting a dead person is an emergency will allow them to obtain a better post-mortem examination. It is indeed necessary to insist on the one hand on the distress of the relatives, whom the doctor will be able to listen to in order to bring comfort. But it is also necessary to move without delay to avoid a death being made up. To this end, it is essential to provide future doctors with the keys to dating the death according to the signs observed. Continuous training, in a constant process of improvement of its practices, would be a precious tool to be set up. One or two training courses per year, providing a credit for continuing medical education, reminding the essential bases of death certification, would certainly make this exercise less arduous and more familiar [35, 37, 45].

The quality of knowledge can be improved even before the end of the university curriculum by offering training in the form of seminars to medical interns and residents, lasting one or two days, based on an interactive and dynamic methodology alternating learning by problem solving, criticism of authentic CMDs, reading of reference articles and finally by proposing a self-assessment by a pre-test and a post-test [44, 46, 47].

Several studies have evaluated the consequences of an educational intervention on doctors practising in hospitals and have found a significant improvement in the quality of writing and a reduction in the percentage of errors. Thus, an Australian study found a 7.3% improvement in the occurrence of errors after training (from 22.4% before to 15.1% after training) [46], the study by Ali et al [48] also showed a significant regression in the occurrence of errors after training workshops (from 92.7% to 40.7% of errors). The study by Myers et al [6] found a decrease in the occurrence of errors after educational intervention with a decrease in the mechanisms of death mentioned, an improvement in the identification of deaths with OML, not using age as a cause of death (prematurity, old age) and the cause of death should be as complete and specific as possible. However, these studies have focused on the short-term effectiveness of these educational interventions and not on the long-term. In summary, the content of such training should be prepared in conjunction with medical, judicial and statistical authorities. The involvement of all the actors in the death certification chain is essential, in order to adjust the content of the courses as well as possible, according to the main errors noted. The form should also be adapted to the audience: lectures, clinical cases or concrete cases. In addition to this training/information, the possibility of having a guide in pocket format, to be able to refer to it in case of difficulty, should be considered [18,37]. In France, aids are available online, notably on the site of the Centre for Epidemiology of Medical Causes of Death. Unfortunately, and this is one of the stumbling blocks of electronic certification, the possibility of connecting to the Internet is not always easy when the doctor is at the bed of the deceased. And even if connectivity via mobile phones is progressing, not all doctors are yet equipped, and network coverage is far from uniform throughout Tunisia. The pocket book format to be slipped into one's bag when the doctor is called to report the death is still the most appropriate format. In our opinion, this guide should contain the following information:

- general recommendations on filling out the certificate, and explain the ultimate purpose of all these check boxes, so that the physician is fully aware of his or her work.
- practical clinical cases, to be able to refer to the most common situations.
- European recommendations on autopsy, or their translation by the National Medical Council in Tunisia.
- a guide to recognizing potentially suspicious situations, especially in cases of suspected suicide. This is to help the physician to differentiate between a suicide and a homicide masquerading as a suicide. Such guides exist in the United States and in some European countries such as Finland [18, 49]. We could possibly draw inspiration from them.

Since any doctor can be called upon to certify a death, it is often the case that the doctor called to the deceased is not his or her own doctor.

Hence the many difficulties reported by certifying doctors in determining the sequence of medical causes of death, especially in elderly people with multiple pathologies. The ideal, but very difficult to achieve, would be to be able to contact the victim's attending physician. In this case, knowledge of the co-morbidities from which the deceased was suffering is a great help in certifying the deaths, as well as in knowing the associated pathologies to be filled out in part II of the certificate. If the doctor is unable to do so, the replacement doctor or another doctor in the department (in the case of a hospital death) must complete the certificate, which will then be countersigned by the doctor in charge. Concerning the OML box, the first recommendation is to write all the practical situations where the OML must be ticked on the back of the CMD, based on the European recommendations [38]. This will greatly facilitate the task of the certifying physician.
In addition to this, a forensic medical service can be introduced, which exists in certain European countries [43]. In this way, the certifying physician could call on this hotline in case of doubt about the death that he has to establish. We also think that this on-call number should be widely distributed. To the different police forces and national guards. The latter would then call in priority doctors trained in body removal. In order to improve the knowledge of the doctors performing the body removal, their participation in the autopsy would be desirable. In this way they could compare their interpretation of the signs they have noted on the corpse with the results of the autopsy.
Another proposal, already practised in France, is the introduction of the registrar. This function generates a great deal of experience in the certification of deaths. This doctor would therefore be particularly capable of recognizing suspicious deaths, and would then call in the forensic doctors. The main disadvantage of this position lies in the fact that this doctor would be unaware of the deceased and his previous state of health [18].
As for the heading "mise en bière", it concerns contagious or epidemic diseases. In our Tunisian model, the diseases that require immediate burial are contagious, epidemic or infectious diseases such as cholera, rabies, viral hepatitis except hepatitis A and viral hemorrhagic fevers. This list has not yet been amended to include COVID 19 infection.

4.2. Concerning modifications to be considered on the certificate

In Tunisia, our model of CMD seems acceptable, especially with the new model (Appendix 2). In France, all the doctors questioned were in favour of mentioning the European recommendations on autopsy on the death certificate [18]. 18] They consider that this would help them in their arguments with the police and the families. The fact that this is written on an official document would give them more weight in the face of the pressure they feel when writing the certificate.
Sometimes, the estimation of the date and time of death was difficult, especially in the case of advanced putrefaction for example. For this purpose, it would be useful to create an additional box to differentiate the estimated date and time of death from the date and time of arrival at the scene.
It is also a good idea to write a telephone number and the name of a person who could answer any difficulties encountered by the certifying physician when writing the CMD on the back of the CMD [49].

4.3. Concerning medical death certificates for corpses that have undergone a forensic autopsy:

In several countries, the CMD may be modified after a forensic autopsy in order to rectify the cause of death which is often missing in CMDs received by the forensic service, depending on the results. Indeed, if additional medical information or autopsy results are available that may lead to a change in the cause of death reported at the beginning, the original death certificate must be modified by the certifying physician by immediately reporting the revised cause of death by making a new CMD. As for the missing certificates, some are most certainly filed with the other court documents after the family has given them to the OPJ. Far from blaming the OPJ or the magistrates investigating the cases, information explaining the "normal" circuit of the death certificate would certainly improve the return of these documents to the Ministry of Health in an anonymous manner. Especially since this document, sealed by the coroner, is of no use in the procedure, since the magistrate also has the autopsy report, which is much more detailed than the simple death certificate [18].

CONCLUSIONS

The medical death certificate is not only a civil status document but also a social and medico-legal document and a source of epidemiological data. It has been adopted by Tunisia since 1999 and is issued by a doctor. This document is essential for the declaration of death to the civil status services before any funeral operations. The certifying physician may be held liable on the basis of what he notes on the medical death certificate. The objectives of our work were to study the content of medical death certificates, to evaluate the quality of writing and to analyse major and minor writing errors. Our work consisted of a prospective descriptive study, extended over a period of 12 months from January 2020 to December 2020, including all medical death certificates received at the Forensic Medicine Department of Habib Bourguiba Hospital in Sfax. During the study period, we collected 74 medical death certificates meeting the inclusion criteria. Concerning the administrative part, nine socio-demographic parameters were studied. The majority of the criteria were met. This result was consistent with the literature where this section was completed at around 92%. The complete identification of the physician was satisfactory in more than 60% of the cases, including his signature and stamp. This result was consistent with the Lebanese and Sudanese study where these data were present in 50% and 82%. The four boxes for medico-legal data (date, time of death, burial, medico-legal obstacle) were completed in more than 90% of the death certificates. When the doctor did not know the date and time of death, he could either give an approximate date or the date and time of discovery of the corpse. The list of illnesses for the heading of the coffin should be revised to include other pathologies and, why not, cases of highly decomposed corpses. Concerning the medical section, and although confidentiality in death certificates was a legal and ethical obligation, doctors only sealed this section in two thirds of the cases. This result was similar to the result of the French study (75%), which attributed this to an oversight, to the state of the medical death certificate and to a reluctance on the part of doctors to lick the self-adhesive part, which, moreover, should be replaced by self-adhesive strips. Some countries, such as the Netherlands, have proposed sending the two parts of the medical certificate of death separately. The drafting of the part concerning the causes of death was at the origin of almost all the drafting errors. We classified these errors into six major ones: only the mechanism of death was mentioned (absence of the cause of death), the sequence of causes of death was incorrect, the cause of death was insufficient, several causes of death were mentioned, the cause of death was unacceptable, and the box "presence of medico-legal obstacle" was not checked. Our classification was inspired by the different classifications reported in the literature. The percentage of medical death certificates without major errors was 17.6%, far behind the Taiwanese, English and Irish studies, but better than the Indian, Pakistani, American and South African studies. The frequency of major errors varied between 33% and 60% depending on the study and in all cases was lower than in our study. The most frequent major error in the different studies was the mention of the mechanism of death without the cause of death, varying between 7% and 47% (5.8% in our study). The most frequent mechanisms of death were: cardiopulmonary arrest, multivisceral failure, shock, sepsis... this was explained by the fact that most physicians tended to confuse causes of death with mechanisms of death. The sixth major fault was when the box for medico-legal impediment to burial was not ticked. This box had to be checked in cases of violent death (accident, suicide, homicide), suspicious death and sudden death. This is an error which has serious consequences, particularly in legal matters (possible involvement of a third party in the death). To facilitate the task of the certifying physician, we recommend that all the circumstances requiring a medico-legal autopsy be written on the back of our model death certificate, based on the European recommendations concerning the harmonisation of rules on medico-legal autopsies. As for minor errors, the absence of a time interval between the onset of the disease and the occurrence of death was the most frequent error in the literature, between 35% and 92%. It could be explained by the lack of attention paid by certifying physicians to this item. In our study, the most frequent error was the use of abbreviations. In some situations, the nosologist was unable to decipher the abbreviation or sometimes misinterpreted it. In Tunisia, as elsewhere in the world, a practical guide for writing the medical death certificate has been developed. In this guide, the rules of writing are well specified and illustrated by examples and practical cases. This national guide was developed in 1998 but our work has shown that an additional effort should be made to improve the quality of the writing. To this end, we have proposed a number of recommendations concerning, in particular

- The training which, until now, has remained insufficient knowing that the medical student receives only one hour and a half of theoretical teaching on the medical certificate of death and this within the framework of the certificate of Legal Medicine taught in 5th year. We offer training in the form of one or two-day seminars to medical interns and residents, based on an interactive and dynamic methodology alternating learning by problem solving, criticism of authentic death certificates, reading of reference articles and finally by proposing a self-assessment by a pre-test and a post-test. These interactive workshops have proven their effectiveness in the United States, Australia and England where the percentage of errors has been reduced by half after an educational intervention.

- The preparation of final death certificates after autopsy to correct the cause of death based on autopsy and/or post-mortem findings.

- The mention of all the practical situations where the medico-legal obstacle must be ticked off on the back of the medical death certificate, based on the European recommendations. This will greatly facilitate the task of the certifying physician.

Despite the various shortcomings of our study, particularly the small sample size, it could be a starting point for several other more complete and broader studies. Finally, the doctor must not forget that the writing of a death certificate is a medical act as important as the care given to the patients and also that it is a serious act because it risks to engage his responsibility and he must write it in all prudence.

REFERENCES

1. Vallin J, Mesl F. Les causes de décès en France de 1925 à 1978. Paris: Institut national d'études démographiques : Presses universitaires de France, 1988.

2. Republic of Tunisia. Decree n°99-1043 of 17 May 1999 fixing the model of the medical certificate of death and the mentions it must contain. Journal Officiel de la République Tunisienne, 28 May 1999; 43:815-818.

3. Lu TH, Shau WY, Shih TP, Lee MC, Chou MC, Lin CK. Factors associated with errors in death certificate completion. A national study in Taiwan. J Clin Epidemiol. 2001;54(3):232-8.

4. Burger EH, Van der Merwe L, Volmink J. Errors in the completion of the death notification form. S Afr Med J. 2007;97(11):1077-81.

5. Katsakiori PF, Panagiotopoulou EC, Sakellaropoulos GC, Papazafiropoulou A, Kardara M. Errors in death certificates in a rural area of Greece. Rural Remote Health. 2007;7(4):822.

6. Myers KA, Farquhar DRE. Improving the accuracy of death certification. Can Med Assoc J. 1998;158:1317-23.

7. Slater DN. Certifying the cause of death: an audit of wording inaccuracies. J Clin Pathol. 1993;46:232-4.

8. Armour A, Bharucha H. Nosological inaccuracies in death certification in Northern Ireland. Ulster Med J. 1997;66:13-7.

9. Canas F, Lorin De La Grandmaison G, Guillou PJ, Jeunehomme G, Durigon M, Bernard
MH. The medico-legal obstacle in the death certificate. Rev Prat. 2005;55:587-94.

10. Manaouil C, Montpellier D. Some practical information about the death certificate. Ann Fr Anesth Reanim. 2008;27:186-9.

11. Stark MM. Literature review of death certification procedures - international aspects. J Clin Forensic Med. 2003;10(1):21-6.

12. Maatoug J, Jedidi M, Ben Dhiab M, Harrabi I, Ghannem H, Zemni M, et al. Death certificates and mortality statistics: comparison between Tunisia and France. In: Duguet AM, ed. Access to organ and tissue transplantation in Europe and rights to care in Europe. Bordeaux: Les Études Hospitalières; 2009. p. 303-10.

13. Republic of Tunisia. Law No. 57-3 of 1 August 1957 regulating civil status. Official Gazette of the Tunisian Republic of 2 August 1957;3:10-16.

14. Tunisian Republic. Decree n° 97-1326 of July 7, 1997 relating to the modalities of preparation of graves and fixing the rules of burial and exhumation of mortal remains or corpses. Journal Officiel de la République Tunisienne, 22 July 1997;58:1279-80.

15. Torres E, Couessurel N. What is a death certificate? Generalist. 2001;2158:112.

16. Khemekhem Z, Hammami Z, Ayadi A, Bardaa S, Maatoog S. Legislative and regulatory aspects of death in Tunisia. JIM Sfax. 2008;15/16:4-7.

17. Republic of Tunisia. Decree No. 81-1634 of 30 November 1981 on the general internal regulations of hospitals, institutes and specialized centres under the Ministry of Public Health. Journal Officiel de la République Tunisienne of 4 December 1981;77: 2831-37.

18. El Nour A, Ibrahim Y, Ali M. Evaluation of death certificates in the pediatric hospitals in Khartoum state during 2004. Sudan J Public Health. 2007; 2(1):29-37.

19. Haque AS, Shamim K, Siddiqui NH, Irfan M, Khan JA. Death certificate completion skills of hospital physicians in a developing country. BMC Health Services Research. 2013;13:205.

20. Swift B, West K. Death certification: an audit of practice entering the 21st century. J Clin Pathol. 2002;55:275-9.

21. Sibai AM, Nuwayhid I, Beydoun M, Chaaya M. Inadequacies of death certification in Beirut: Who is responsible? Bulletin of the World Health Organization. 2002;80(7):555-61.

22. U.S. Department of Health and Human Services, Center for Disease Control and Prevention. Physicians' Handbook on Medical Certification of Death [Online]. National Center for Health Statistics, April 2003. [cited 2013-03-14];[about 65 screens]. Available from URL: http://www.cdc.gov/nchs/data/misc/hb_cod.pdf

23. Epain D. Medical certificates and emergencies - assault and battery certificates. EMC- Medicine. 2005;2(4):448-67.

24. Manaouil C, Decourcelle M, Gignon M, Chatelain D, Jardé O. The death certificate: how to fill it in and why? Ann Fr Anesth Reanim. 2007;26:434-9.

25. Tunisian Republic. Code of medical ethics: official printing house of the Tunisian Republic 2006.

26. Tunisian Republic. Tunisian Penal Code. Official Printing Office of the Tunisian Republic 2013.

27. Quantitative and qualitative assessment of the notification of deaths and the reporting of their causes (Number and quality of completion of death certificates [Online]. Institut National de Santé Publique [cited 20/02/2013];[about 5 screens]. Available from URL: http://www.insp.nat.tn/fr/cause_dece/programme_national.html

28. Office of the Registrar General. Handbook on medical certification of death [Online]. Ministry of Consumer and Business Services, August 2010 [cited 24/02/2014] Available from URL: http://www.publications.serviceontario.ca/ecomlinks/016600.pdf

29. U.S. Department of Health and Human Services, Center for Disease Control and Prevention. Instruction Manual. Part 20: ICD-10 cause of death querying 2010 [Online]. National Center for Health Statistics, December 2009 [cited 2014/01/27] Available from URL: http://www.cdc.gov/nchs/data/dvs/20_Instruction_Manual_2010.pdf

30. Agarwal S, Kumar V, Kumar L, Bastia BK, Chavali KH. A study on appraisal of effectiveness of the MCCD scheme. J Indian Acad Forensic Med. 2010;32(4):318-20.

31. Quantitative and qualitative assessment of the notification of deaths and the declaration of their causes (Number and quality of completion of death certificates [Online]. InstitutNationaldeSantéPublique[cited 20/02/2013]. Available from: http://www.insp.nat.tn/fr/cause_dece/programme_national.html

32. Hajem S, Hsairi M. The national system of information on causes of death: diagnosis of the situation and main results. Revue Tunisienne de Santé Publique 2013;1:7-23.

33. Bouafif N, Hajem S, Ennigrou S, Touati M, Ben Hamida A, Zouari B. Declaration of causes of death in Tunisia. Tunis Med. 2000;78(12):713-718.

34. Cheng TJ, Lee FC, Lin SJ, Lu TH. Improper cause-of-death statements by specialty of certifying physician: a cross-sectional study in two medical centres in Taiwan. BMJ Open [Online]. 2013 February [10/02/2013];2(4):[7 pages]. Available from URL: http://bmjopen.bmj.com/content/2/4/e001229.long

35. Pritt BS, Hardin NJ, Richmond JA, Shapiro SL. Death certification errors at an academic institution. Arch Pathol Lab Med. 2005;129(11):1476-9.

36. Jordan JM, Bass MJ. Errors in death certificate completion in a teaching hospital. Clin Invest Med. 1993;16(4):249-55.

37. Abadie AL. Analysis of ill-defined and unknown causes of death in metropolitan France in 2009. Study and proposals for improving death certification [Thesis]. Doctorate in Medicine: Paris; 2012. 122p.

38. Vial-Reyt K, Vallée J. Death certification and general practitioners: opinions on proposals for improvement (qualitative survey of 14 general practitioners in the Loire). Rev Prat. 2011;61:1401-10.

39. Tunisian Republic. Law n°75-33 of 14/05/1975 promulgating the organic law of communes. Journal Officiel de la République Tunisienne of 20 May 1975;34:1056-64.

40. Chatelain D, Manaouil C, Manaouil D, Regimbeau JM. Autopsies and surgical services. Ann Chir. 2005;130:212-7.

41. Patel AB, Rathod H, Rana H, Patel V. Assessment of medical certificate of cause of death at a new teaching hospital in Vadodara. National Journal of Community Medicine. 2011;2(3);349-53.

42. Pandya H, Bose N, Shah R, Chaudhury N, Phatak A. Educational intervention to improve death certification at a teaching hospital. Natl Med J India. 2009;22:317-19.

43. Peach HG, Brumley DJ. Death certification by doctors in non-metropolitan Victoria. Aust Fam Physician. 1998;27:178-82.

44. Degani AT, Patel RM, Smith BE, Grimsley E. The effect of student training on accuracy of completion of death certificates. Med Educ Online [Online]. September 2009 [29/01/2014];14(17):[5 pages]. Available from URL: http://med-ed

online.net/index.php/meo/article/view/4510

45. Villar J, Pérez-Méndez L. Evaluating an educational intervention to improve the accuracy of death certification among trainees from various specialties. BMC Health Services Research. 2007;7:183.

46. Weeramanthri T, Beresford W, Sathianathan V. An evaluation of an educational intervention to improve death certification practice. Aust Clin Rev. 1993;13(4):185-9.

47. Pieterse D, Groenewald P, Bradshaw D, Burger EH, Rohde J, Reagon G. Death Certificates: Let's Get It Right. S Afr Med J. 2009;99(9):643-4.

48. Ali NMA, Hamadeh RR. Improving the Accuracy of Death Certification among Secondary Care Physicians. Bahrain Medical Bulletin [Online]. 2013 June [30/01/2014];35(2):[6 pages]. Available from URL: http://www.bahrainmedicalbulletin.com/june_2013/Improving_Accuracy.pdf

49. U.S. Department of Health and Human Services, Center for Disease Control and Prevention. Medical Examiners' and Coroners' Handbook on Death Registration and Featal Death Reporting [Online]. National Center for Health Statistics, April 2003 [cited 12/02/2014]; [approximately 138 screens]. Available from URL: http://www.cdc.gov/nchs/data/misc/hb_me.pdf

50. Pavillon G, Laurent F. Certification and coding of medical causes of death. Bull Epidemiol Hebd. 2003;30-31:134-8.

51. Pavillon G, Coilland P, Jougla E. Implementation of electronic certification of medical causes of death in France: initial assessment and prospects. Bull Epidemiol Hebd. 2007;35-36:306-8.

ANNEXES

Appendix 1: DEATH CERTIFICATE EVALUATION SHEET

File No. :

THE UPPER PART		YES	NO
1. DEFUNT: Has he registered his :			
Full name:			
Exact identity or not			
CIN number :			
Address: Governorate:			
Date of birth or age: Age:			
Sex: M: F :			
Profession:			
Marital status:			
Nationality:			
Place of death: Governorate:			
Number of criteria met:/9			
2. PHYSICIAN: Did he/she mention his/her :			
Name:			
Physician's Specialty:	Mention :		
Grade:	Mention :		
CNOM registration number :			
Location of practice:	CHU- HR-HC- MLP- Governorate:		
Is it the attending physician?			
Signature and stamp :			

To whom is the certificate issued, is it mentioned?		
Number of criteria met: /7		
3. FORENSIC DATA :		
Date of death mentioned		
Time of death reported		
Is there a forensic barrier?		
Is the box for "committal" checked?		
Number of criteria met in the upper part: /20		
THE LOWER PART		
Is it sealed? :		
1. Medical data		
Number of lines filled:/4		
Causes of death mentioned :		
Mechanism of death mentioned :		
Initial cause mentioned:		
Immediate cause mentioned :		
The causal hierarchy is respected:		
The time frame of the morbid states is noted:		
Are other morbid conditions contributing to the death mentioned? (II):		
2. Additional information:		
A current pregnancy (if any) is mentioned:		
A delivery within the last year:		
If the cause is an accident, is the exact location mentioned?		
If the cause is an accident at work; is this entity mentioned?		

The exact place of death is mentioned:			
Is the box concerning the autopsy checked?			
Does the certificate comply with the model decree No. 99 ?			
Numberof major errors:/ 6	1. Only the mechanism of death is mentioned		
	2. The sequence of causes of death is incorrect		
	3. The cause of death is insufficient		
	4. Several causes of death are mentioned		
	5. The cause of death is unacceptable		
	6. The box "presence of medical/legal barriers" is not checked		

TABLE OF CONTENTS

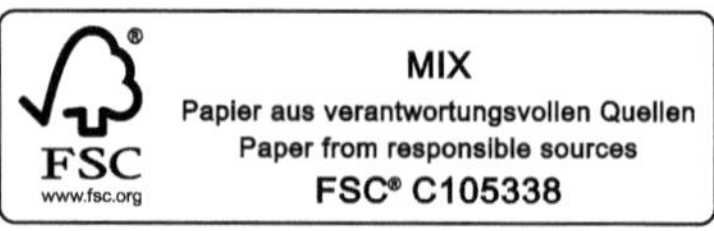

Printed by Books on Demand GmbH, Norderstedt / Germany